Congestive Heart Failure Cookbook For Seniors

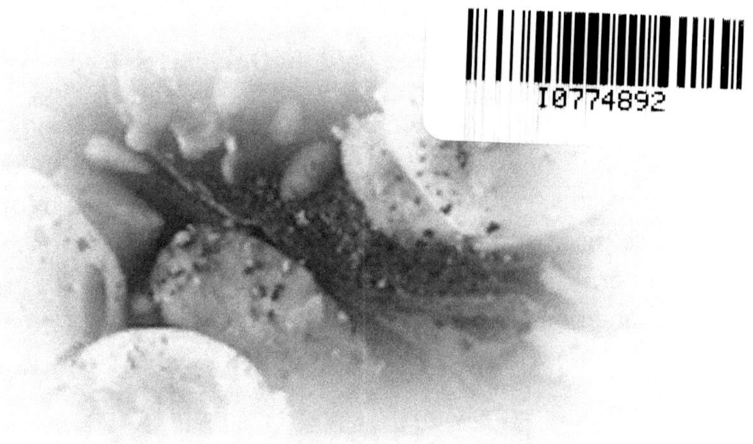

Comprehensive Guide to Healthy and Nutritious Recipes for Improving your Heart Health

David T. Salcedo

CHECK OTHER RELATED BOOKS

LOW SODIUM COOKBOOK FOR CONGESTIVE HEART FAILURE

TABLE OF CONTENTS

INTRODUCTION

Sarah, a vibrant 65-year-old woman who discovered her path to wellness after being diagnosed with Congestive Heart Failure (CHF). Sarah accepted the challenge with tenacity and resilience, rather than abandoning herself to a life of restrictions.

Sarah's adventure began with a visit to her cardiologist, where she was diagnosed with CHF. She was shocked and worried about her health, so she decided it was time to take charge. Her doctor emphasized the importance of diet in managing CHF, with a special emphasis on lowering blood pressure and cholesterol levels.

As she went into the area of heart-healthy food, Sarah encountered a steep learning curve. She changed her eating habits to include more fresh, nutrient-dense foods. Her kitchen was transformed, with salt alternatives, nutritious grains, and an assortment of bright fruits and vegetables taking center stage.

Sarah walked through the grocery store aisles with a fresh viewpoint. She learned to read food labels, spot hidden sodium, and make educated decisions. As she discovered heart-healthy choices and fresh vegetables to feed her body, her trip to the grocery became a powerful experience.

Sarah improved her kitchen after gaining knowledge. She experimented with herbs and spices, creating delectable combinations that added taste without the need for salt. Her kitchen became a health sanctuary, creating a pleasant environment for her transforming path.

Sarah set out on a culinary journey, seeking out heart-healthy foods that satisfied her taste buds while also matching with her new nutritional goals. She realized that eating for heart health could be both enjoyable and gratifying, with anything from vivid salads to lean protein-packed meals.

Sarah understood she wasn't alone on her adventure. She sought help from friends, relatives, and online forums. Sharing recipes, stories, and words of support became an important part of her healing journey.

Sarah integrated mild exercises into her program after realizing the value of a holistic approach. She engaged in hobbies such as walking, yoga, and gardening, which improved her cardiovascular health and overall well-being.

Sarah kept track of her blood pressure and cholesterol levels as she committed to her new lifestyle. Her commitment to remain on this transforming road was strengthened by witnessing favorable developments.

Every minor win became reason for celebration. Sarah acknowledged and celebrated her victories, whether it was reaching a weight loss goal or creating a new heart-healthy recipe, reinforcing her commitment to a heart-healthy lifestyle.

OVERVIEW OF CONGESTIVE HEART FAILURE (CHF)

Congestive Heart Failure is a chronic condition in which the heart is unable to adequately pump blood, resulting in an insufficient supply of oxygen to fulfill the body's needs.

Overview

CHF is caused by the heart muscle weakening or stiffening, reducing its capacity to fill or evacuate blood.

The condition frequently causes fluid buildup, which causes congestion in the lungs and other tissues.

Types of Congestive Heart Failure

Systolic Heart Failure

Description: Impaired heart muscle contraction.

Characteristics: Characteristics include a lower ejection fraction, which is the amount of blood pushed out of the heart during each contraction.

Diastolic Heart Failure

Description: Impaired heart muscle relaxation.

Characteristics: Features include a preserved ejection fraction but difficulty filling with blood during the resting phase.

Right-Sided Heart Failure

Description: Impaired right ventricle function.

Manifestations: Peripheral edema (swelling), hepatomegaly, and ascites.

Left-Sided Heart Failure

Description: Impaired left ventricle function.

Manifestations: Pulmonary congestion, shortness of breath, and fatigue.

Causes of Congestive Heart Failure

Coronary Artery Disease (CAD)

Atherosclerosis and myocardial infarction both contribute to heart muscle weakness.

Hypertension (High Blood Pressure)

Chronic pressure overload causes cardiac damage and may result in heart failure.

Cardiomyopathies

Heart muscle structural defects that are either genetic or acquired.

Valvular Heart Disease

Heart valve dysfunction has an impact on cardiac function.

Other Contributing Factors

Diabetes, cardiovascular infections, and substance abuse.

Symptoms of Congestive Heart Failure

Common Clinical Manifestations

- Shortness of breath (dyspnea)

- Fatigue and weakness

- Swelling (edema) in extremities

- Persistent coughing and wheezing

- Fluid retention and weight gain

Severity and Progression

CHF progresses through stages, with symptoms worsening over time.

Preventive Measures for Congestive Heart Failure

Lifestyle Modifications

- Adopting a heart-healthy diet (low in sodium, saturated fats).
- Regular exercise and physical activity.
- Weight management and obesity prevention.

Blood Pressure Management

- Regular monitoring of blood pressure levels.
- Adherence to prescribed medications and treatment plans.

Cardiac Rehabilitation

- Post-myocardial infarction recovery through exercise, education, and support.

Early Detection and Treatment of Risk Factors

- Management of diabetes and other contributing conditions.
- Timely intervention for valvular heart disease.

PREVALENCE AMONG SENIORS

Congestive Heart Failure (CHF) is common in the elderly due to a combination of age-related changes in the cardiovascular system, the cumulative effect of risk factors over time, and the presence of comorbidities. Here are some of the major factors that contribute to the occurrence of CHF among seniors:

Age-Related Changes

Reduced Cardiac Reserve: As we age, our hearts' ability to respond to stress and effort decreases. The heart may become less efficient at pumping blood, resulting in decreased cardiac reserve and making elders more vulnerable to heart failure.

Stiffening of Arteries: As we age, our arteries lose their suppleness, resulting to increasing resistance to blood flow. This can result in increased blood pressure and strain on the heart.

Changes in Heart Structure: As we age, structural changes such as thickening of the heart walls and valves can develop. These changes can reduce the effectiveness of the heart's pumping and contribute to heart failure.

Cumulative Impact of Risk Factors

Long-Term Exposure: Seniors may have a longer history of risk factor exposure, such as hypertension, diabetes, and high cholesterol. The cumulative effect of these factors over time can raise the risk of getting CHF.

Lifestyle Factors: Unhealthy lifestyle behaviors like poor food, sedentary behavior, and smoking can become ingrained over time. These behaviors contribute to the onset and progression of cardiovascular illnesses that lead to CHF.

Comorbidities

High Prevalence of Chronic Conditions: Seniors are prone to many chronic disorders such as hypertension, diabetes, and coronary artery disease. These diseases contribute significantly to the development of CHF and create a complex health landscape.

Interconnected Health Issues: Comorbidities can exacerbate each other, causing a cascade effect that pressures the cardiovascular system and raises the risk of heart failure.

THE IMPORTANCE OF DIETARY MANAGEMENT IN CONGESTIVE HEART FAILURE

Dietary management plays a pivotal role in the overall care and well-being of individuals with Congestive Heart Failure (CHF). Here are key reasons highlighting the importance of dietary management:

1. **Control of Sodium Intake**

Fluid Retention Control: Sodium can contribute to fluid retention, causing congestion in the lungs and extremities. Controlling salt consumption is critical for maintaining fluid balance and decreasing symptoms such as edema and shortness of breath.

Blood Pressure Regulation: Sodium has an immediate effect on blood pressure. Dietary management aids in salt control, which is critical for treating hypertension, a primary cause of CHF.

2. **Maintenance of Fluid Balance**

Edema Prevention: Proper dietary control, including fluid intake monitoring, helps to prevent excessive fluid accumulation, lowering the risk of edema and its related consequences.

Heart Function Support: Maintaining an optimal fluid balance is critical for maintaining the heart's ability to efficiently pump blood. Excess fluid can put strain on the heart and aggravate CHF symptoms.

3. **Blood Sugar Management**

Impact on Diabetes: Dietary management is critical for persons with coexisting diabetes in order to keep blood sugar levels stable. This improves overall cardiovascular health and lowers the chance of problems.

KEY NUTRIENTS FOR HEART HEALTH

Maintaining heart health entails not only limiting certain dietary components, but also maintaining enough consumption of vital nutrients that promote cardiovascular health. Here are some vital nutrients, each with a distinct role to play in boosting heart health:

1. Sodium

Role in Heart Health

Sodium is an electrolyte that aids in the regulation of fluid balance within and around cells, particularly those in the heart.

Importance in Heart Health

Excess salt consumption has been related to high blood pressure, a major risk factor for heart disease and Congestive Heart Failure (CHF).

Dietary management incorporating lower sodium intake aids in blood pressure control, reducing the load on the heart.

Sources

High sodium foods include processed and packaged foods, canned soups, processed meats, and restaurant/fast food.

2. Potassium

Role in Heart Health

Potassium is a mineral that is necessary for optimal cardiac rhythm and muscle function.

Importance in Heart Health

Adequate potassium intake helps to regulate blood pressure by offsetting the detrimental effects of sodium.

It helps to maintain electrolyte balance, which is essential for heart function.

Sources

Potassium is abundant in fruits (particularly bananas, oranges, and melons), vegetables (particularly potatoes and spinach), dairy products, and legumes.

3. Fiber

Role in Heart Health

Dietary fiber, including soluble fiber, aids in cholesterol reduction by binding to and eliminating cholesterol from the body.

Importance in Heart Health

Lowering cholesterol lowers the risk of atherosclerosis, which is linked to heart disease.

Fiber also helps with weight loss and enhances overall cardiovascular health.

Sources

Whole grains, fruits, vegetables, nuts, and seeds are high in dietary fiber.

4. Omega-3 Fatty Acids

Role in Heart Health

Omega-3 fatty acids, such as EPA and DHA (docosahexaenoic acid), have anti-inflammatory and anti-arrhythmic properties.

Importance in Heart Health

Omega-3 fatty acids promote heart health by lowering triglyceride levels, blood pressure, and preventing irregular heartbeats.

They also improve blood vessel function and reduce inflammation, which contributes to overall cardiovascular health.

Sources

Omega-3 fatty acids are abundant in fatty fish (salmon, mackerel, sardines), flaxseeds, chia seeds, walnuts, and algae-based supplements.

5. Magnesium

Role in Heart Health

Magnesium is required for proper muscle and neuron function, including heart muscle.

Importance in Heart Health

Adequate magnesium levels promote blood vessel function and assist sustain a regular heartbeat.

A lack of magnesium has been related to an increased risk of heart disease and CHF.

Sources

Foods high in magnesium include leafy green vegetables, nuts, seeds, whole grains, and legumes.

FOOD TO EAT AND FOOD TO AVOID

Foods to Eat for Heart Health

1. Fruits and Vegetables

Berries, citrus fruits, leafy greens, tomatoes, and cruciferous vegetables are good sources of vitamins, minerals, fiber, and antioxidants.

2. Whole Grains

Fiber, B vitamins, and minerals are found in brown rice, quinoa, oats, whole wheat, and barley.

3. Fatty Fish

Salmon, mackerel, trout, and sardines are high in omega-3 fatty acids, which are beneficial to heart health.

4. Nuts and Seeds

Almonds, walnuts, chia seeds, and flaxseeds are high in healthful fats, fiber, and nutrients.

5. Legumes

Examples is said to include chickpeas, beans and lentils which are high in protein, fiber, and potassium.

6. **Lean Proteins**

Skinless poultry, lean cuts of beef or pork, and plant-based protein sources such as tofu and tempeh help to maintain a heart-healthy diet.

7. **Dairy or Dairy Alternatives**

Calcium and vitamin D are found in low-fat or fat-free yogurt, milk, and fortified plant-based milk alternatives.

8. **Healthy Fats**

Avocados, olive oil, and canola oil are high in monounsaturated fats, which are good for your heart.

9. **Herbs and Spices**

Garlic, ginger, turmeric, and other herbs and spices can provide flavor without adding too much sodium.

10. **Dark Chocolate**

Dark chocolate with at least 70% cocoa content includes antioxidants and may have heart-protective advantages when consumed in moderation.

Foods to Limit or Avoid

1. High-Sodium Foods

Processed meals, canned soups, fast food, and salty snacks can all raise blood pressure.

2. Trans Fats

Limit or avoid items that include partly hydrogenated oils, which are commonly found in margarines, fried foods, and processed snacks.

3. Saturated Fats

Limiting your diet of saturated fats, which are found in fatty meats, full-fat dairy products, and some oils, will help you manage your cholesterol levels.

4. Added Sugars

It is critical for overall heart health to limit sugary beverages, candies, and processed foods with added sugars.

5. **Excess Red and Processed Meats**

A high intake of red and processed meats is linked to an increased risk of heart disease. Select lean protein sources and limit your intake.

6. **Highly Processed Foods**

Highly processed foods are frequently high in harmful fats, salt, and added sugars. Choose whole, minimally processed options.

7. **Excessive Alcohol**

While moderate alcohol consumption may have cardiovascular benefits, excessive alcohol consumption might have a negative impact on health. It is critical to restrict alcohol usage.

8. **Sugar-Sweetened Beverages**

Sugary fruit juices, sodas, and energy drinks can all contribute to weight gain and have a bad influence on heart health. Instead, choose for water, herbal tea, or unsweetened beverages.

9. **Full-Fat Dairy**

To lower saturated fat intake, limit high-fat dairy products and opt for low-fat or fat-free alternatives.

10. **Fast Food:**

Fast food is frequently heavy in harmful fats, salt, and calories. To improve heart health, it is best to minimize consumption.

CHAPTER 1

Breakfast Recipes

1. Berry-licious Oatmeal with Chia Seeds & Nuts

Ingredients

- 1/2 cup rolled oats
- 1 cup unsweetened almond milk
- 1/2 cup mixed berries
- 1 tbsp chia seeds
- 1/4 cup chopped walnuts
- 1/4 tsp cinnamon
- Honey (optional)

Preparation

1. Simmer oats and almond milk in a saucepan until thickened.

2. Stir in berries, chia seeds, and cinnamon.

3. Let sit for 5 minutes to thicken.

4. Top with walnuts and drizzle with honey if desired.

Nutritional Information

- 240 calories
- 5g fat
- 35g carbs
- 8g protein
- 4g fiber
- 150mg sodium

Serving Size: 1 cup

Prep Time: 10 minutes

2. Smoked Salmon & Avocado Whole-Wheat Toast
Ingredients

- 1 slice whole-wheat toast

- 1/4 avocado, sliced

- 2 oz smoked salmon

- 1 tbsp low-fat cream cheese

- Lemon juice

- Black pepper

Preparation

1.   Toast bread.

2.   Mash avocado on toast.

3.   Top with smoked salmon, cream cheese, lemon juice, and black pepper.

Nutritional Information

- 250 calories

- 10g fat

- 25g carbs

- 15g protein

- 3g fiber

- 250mg sodium

Serving Size: 1 slice

Prep Time: 5 minutes

3. Spinach & Egg Scramble with Tomatoes

Ingredients

- 1 cup spinach

- 2 eggs

- 1/4 cup chopped tomatoes

- 1/4 tsp olive oil

- Salt

- Pepper

Preparation

1. Heat olive oil in a pan.

2. Add spinach and cook until wilted.

3. Push spinach to one side, pour in eggs, and scramble.

4. Stir in tomatoes, salt, and pepper.

Nutritional Information

- 150 calories

- 5g fat

- 10g carbs

- 12g protein

- 2g fiber

- 150mg sodium

Serving Size: 1 cup

Prep Time: 10 minutes

4. Greek Yogurt Parfait with Berries & Granola

Ingredients

- 1/2 cup plain Greek yogurt

- 1/2 cup mixed berries

- 1/4 cup granola

- Honey (optional)

Preparation

1.   Layer yogurt, berries, and granola in a parfait glass.

2.   Drizzle with honey if desired.

Nutritional Information

- 200 calories

- 5g fat

- 25g carbs

- 15g protein

- 3g fiber

- 150mg sodium

Serving Size: 1 cup

Prep Time: 5 minutes

5. Smoothie Bowl with Spinach, Banana & Peanut Butter

Ingredients

- 1 cup spinach

- 1 banana

- 1/2 cup unsweetened almond milk

- 1 tbsp peanut butter

- 1/4 tsp flaxseeds

- Cinnamon

Preparation

1.   Blend spinach, banana, almond milk, peanut butter, flaxseeds, and cinnamon until smooth.

2.   Pour into a bowl and top with additional berries or nuts if desired.

Nutritional Information

- 300 calories

- 10g fat

- 40g carbs

- 10g protein

- 5g fiber

- 150mg sodium

Serving Size: 1 bowl

Prep Time: 5 minutes

6. Cottage Cheese & Fruit Toast

Ingredients

- 1 slice whole-wheat toast

- 1/4 cup low-fat cottage cheese

- 1/4 cup sliced fruit (e.g., mango, strawberries)

- Cinnamon

- Honey (optional)

Preparation

1. Toast bread.

2. Spread cottage cheese on toast.

3. Top with fruit, cinnamon, and honey if desired.

Nutritional Information

- 200 calories

- 5g fat

- 25g carbs

- 15g protein

- 1g fiber

- 150mg sodium

Serving Size: 1 slice

Prep Time: 5 minutes

7. Scrambled Tofu with Bell Peppers and Onions

Ingredients

- 1/2 block firm tofu, crumbled

- 1/2 cup chopped bell pepper (any color)

- 1/4 cup chopped onion

- 1/4 tsp turmeric

- 1/4 tsp paprika

- Salt and pepper

- Olive oil spray

Preparation

1. Heat olive oil spray in a pan over medium heat.

2. Add onion and cook until softened.

3. Add bell pepper and cook for another 2-3 minutes.

4.   Crumble tofu into the pan and cook until golden brown, stirring occasionally.

5.   Stir in turmeric and paprika.

6.   Add salt and pepper in order for it to taste

7.   Serve on whole-wheat toast or with a side of fruit.

Nutritional Information

- 200 calories

- 8g fat

- 15g carbs

- 15g protein

- 2g fiber

- 200mg sodium

Serving Size: 1/2 block tofu

Prep Time: 10 minutes

8. Chia Seed Pudding with Berries and Nuts

Ingredients

- 1/4 cup chia seeds

- 1 cup unsweetened almond milk

- 1/4 cup mixed berries

- 1/4 cup chopped nuts (e.g., almonds, walnuts)

- Honey (optional)

Preparation

1.   Combine chia seeds and almond milk in a jar or bowl.

2.   It should be stirred well and refrigerate for at least 2 hours, or overnight.

3.   Top with berries and nuts before serving.

4.   Drizzle with honey if desired.

Nutritional Information

- 250 calories

- 10g fat

- 25g carbs

- 10g protein

- 5g fiber

- 50mg sodium

Serving Size: 1 cup

Prep Time: 5 minutes (plus refrigeration time)

9. Baked Eggs with Avocado and Tomatoes

Ingredients

- 2 eggs

- 1/2 avocado, sliced

- 1/4 cup chopped tomatoes

- Salt and pepper

- Olive oil spray

- Optional toppings: chopped fresh herbs, chili flakes

Preparation

1.   Preheat oven to 400°F (200°C).

2.   Divide avocado slices between two ramekins or oven-safe dishes.

3.   Top each ramekin with tomatoes, egg, salt, and pepper.

4.   Drizzle with olive oil spray.

5.   Bake for 10-12 minutes, or until egg whites are set and yolks are desired consistency.

6.   Top with optional ingredients and serve.

Nutritional Information

- 250 calories

- 15g fat

- 5g carbs

- 12g protein

- 2g fiber

- 150mg sodium

Serving Size: 1 ramekin

Prep Time: 5 minutes

10. Smoothie Bowl with Spinach, Mango, and Coconut

Ingredients

- 1 cup spinach

- 1/2 cup frozen mango chunks

- 1/2 cup unsweetened coconut milk

- 1/4 cup plain Greek yogurt (optional)

- 1/4 tsp ground ginger

- Honey (optional)

Preparation

1.   Blend spinach, mango, coconut milk, yogurt (if using), and ginger until smooth.

2.   Pour into a bowl and top with your favorite toppings, such as shredded coconut, chia seeds, or granola.

3.   Drizzle with honey if desired.

Nutritional Information

- 300 calories

- 10g fat

- 40g carbs

- 10g protein

- 4g fiber

- 80mg sodium

Serving Size: 1 bowl

Prep Time: 5 minutes

11. Sweet Potato Hash with Black Beans and Avocado

Ingredients

- Sweet potato of medium size , peeled and diced

- 1/2 cup black beans, rinsed and drained

- 1/4 cup chopped red onion

- 1/4 cup chopped bell pepper (any color)

- 1/4 tsp chili powder

- 1/4 tsp cumin

- Salt and pepper

- Olive oil spray

- 1/4 avocado, sliced

Preparation

1.   Heat olive oil spray in a skillet over medium heat.

2.   Add sweet potato and cook until softened, about 5-7 minutes.

3.   Add onion and bell pepper and cook until softened, about 3-5 minutes.

4.   Stir in black beans, chili powder, cumin, salt, and pepper.

5.   Cook for another 2-3 minutes, or until heated through.

6.   Serve topped with avocado slices.

Nutritional Information

- 300 calories

- 10g fat

- 40g carbs

- 10g protein

- 5g fiber

- 200mg sodium

Serving Size: 1 serving

Prep Time: 10 minutes

12. Overnight Oats with Berries and Nuts

Ingredients

- 1/2 cup rolled oats

- 1/2 cup unsweetened almond milk

- 1/4 cup mixed berries

- 1/4 cup chopped nuts (e.g., almonds, walnuts)

- 1/4 tsp chia seeds (optional)

- Honey or maple syrup (optional)

Preparation

1.   Combine oats, almond milk, berries, nuts, and chia seeds (if using) in a jar or container.

2.   Stir well and refrigerate overnight.

3.   In the morning, stir before serving and drizzle with honey or maple syrup if desired.

Nutritional Information

- 250 calories

- 10g fat

- 30g carbs

- 10g protein

- 5g fiber

- 50mg sodium

Serving Size: 1 jar or container

Prep Time: 5 minutes (plus refrigeration time)

13. Whole-Wheat Pancakes with Apple and Cinnamon

Ingredients

- 1/2 cup whole-wheat flour

- 1/2 tsp baking powder

- 1/4 tsp cinnamon

- 1/4 cup unsweetened almond milk

- 1/4 cup mashed apple

- 1 egg

- Olive oil spray

- Chopped nuts, berries, maple syrup should be added if you desire it.

Preparation

1.   Whisk together flour, baking powder, and cinnamon in a bowl.

2.   In a separate bowl, whisk together almond milk, mashed apple, and egg.

3.   Wet ingredients and dry ingredients should be added and min until they are thoroughly combined.

4.   Heat olive oil spray in a skillet over medium heat.

5.   Pour batter in 1/4 cup portions and cook until golden brown on both sides, about 2-3 minutes per side.

6.   Serve with your favorite toppings.

Nutritional Information

- 200 calories

- 5g fat

- 30g carbs

- 8g protein

- 2g fiber

- 150mg sodium

Serving Size: 2-3 pancakes

Prep Time: 10 minutes

CHAPTER 2

Lunch Recipes

1. Mediterranean Tuna Salad Sandwich

Ingredients

- 2 cans tuna in water, drained

- 1/2 cup chopped tomatoes

- 1/4 cup chopped cucumber

- 1/4 cup chopped red onion

- 1 tbsp chopped fresh parsley

- 1 tbsp olive oil

- 1 tbsp lemon juice

- Salt and pepper to taste

- 2 slices whole-wheat bread

Preparation

1.   Combine tuna, tomatoes, cucumber, red onion, parsley, olive oil, lemon juice, salt, and pepper in a bowl.

2.   Spread tuna salad on whole-wheat bread and enjoy!

Nutritional Information

- 300 calories

- 10g fat

- 30g carbs

- 25g protein

- 2g fiber

- 300mg sodium

Serving Size: 1 sandwich

Prep Time: 10 minutes

2. Lentil Soup with Whole-Wheat Pita Bread

Ingredients

- 1 cup green lentils, rinsed

- 4 cups vegetable broth

- 1 chopped onion

- 2 chopped carrots

- 2 chopped celery stalks

- 2 cloves garlic, minced

- 1 tsp dried thyme

- 1/2 tsp dried cumin

- Salt and pepper to taste

- Whole-wheat pita bread for dipping

Preparation

1.   Sauté onion, carrots, and celery in a pot with olive oil until softened.

2.   Add lentils, broth, thyme, cumin, salt, and pepper.

3.   It should be brought to a boil then adjust the heat by reducing it and simmer for 30 minutes, or until lentils are tender.

4.   It should be served with whole-wheat pita bread for dipping.

Nutritional Information

- 250 calories
- 5g fat
- 40g carbs
- 15g protein
- 10g fiber
- 350mg sodium

Serving Size: 1 cup soup

Prep Time: 15 minutes

3. Salmon with Roasted Vegetables

Ingredients

- 1 salmon fillet

- 1 tbsp olive oil

- Salt and pepper to taste

- 1 cup chopped broccoli

- 1 cup chopped Brussels sprouts

- 1/2 cup chopped red onion

- 1 clove garlic, minced

Preparation

1.   Preheat oven to 400°F (200°C).

2.   Toss broccoli, Brussels sprouts, red onion, garlic, olive oil, salt, and pepper on a baking sheet.

3.   Roast vegetables for 15-20 minutes, or until tender.

4.   Season salmon with salt and pepper. Place on a separate baking sheet.

5.   Bake salmon for 10-15 minutes, or until cooked through.

6.   Serve salmon with roasted vegetables and enjoy!

Nutritional Information

- 350 calories

- 15g fat

- 20g carbs

- 35g protein

- 5g fiber

- 400mg sodium

Serving Size: 1 salmon fillet and 1/2 cup roasted vegetables

Prep Time: 10 minutes

4. Chicken Caesar Salad with Whole-Wheat Croutons

Ingredients

- 4 oz grilled chicken breast, sliced

- 2 cups romaine lettuce

- 1/2 cup cherry tomatoes, halved

- 1/4 cup grated Parmesan cheese

- 2 tbsp Caesar salad dressing (low-fat)

- 1/4 cup whole-wheat croutons

Preparation

1. Toss romaine lettuce and cherry tomatoes in a bowl.

2. Top with sliced chicken breast, Parmesan cheese, and Caesar dressing.

3. Sprinkle with whole-wheat croutons and enjoy!

Nutritional Information

- 300 calories

- 10g fat

- 20g carbs

- 30g protein

- 2g fiber

- 350mg sodium

- **Serving Size:** 1 salad

- **Prep Time:** 10 minutes

5. Turkey and Avocado Wrap with Sprouts

Ingredients

- 2 whole-wheat tortillas
- 4 oz sliced turkey breast
- 1/2 avocado, sliced
- 1/4 cup alfalfa sprouts
- 1 tbsp Dijon mustard
- 1 tsp lemon juice

Preparation

1.   Spread Dijon mustard and lemon juice on each tortilla.

2.   Top with turkey breast, avocado, and sprouts.

3.   Roll up tortillas and enjoy!

Nutritional Information

- 350 calories

- 15g fat

- 30g carbs

- 20g protein

- 5g fiber

- 300mg sodium

Serving Size: 1 wrap

Prep Time: 5 minutes

6. Black Bean and Corn Salad with Cilantro

Ingredients

- 1 can black beans, drained and rinsed

- 1 cup frozen corn, thawed

- 1/2 cup chopped red onion

- 1/4 cup chopped fresh cilantro

- 1 tbsp olive oil

- 1 tbsp lime juice

- Salt and pepper to taste

Preparation

1.   Combine black beans, corn, red onion, cilantro, olive oil, lime juice, salt, and pepper in a bowl.

2.   Toss to combine and enjoy!

Nutritional Information

- 200 calories

- 5g fat

- 30g carbs

- 10g protein

- 5g fiber

- 150mg sodium

Serving Size: 1 cup salad

Prep Time: 5 minutes

7. Baked Potato with Tuna Salad and Spinach

Ingredients

- 1 medium baked potato

- 2 cans tuna in water, drained

- 1/4 cup chopped celery

- 1/4 cup chopped red onion

- 2 tbsp Greek yogurt

- 1 tbsp lemon juice

- 1 tsp Dijon mustard

- 1/4 cup chopped fresh spinach

- Salt and pepper to taste

Preparation

1.	Bake potato until tender.

2.	Combine tuna, celery, red onion, Greek yogurt, lemon juice, Dijon mustard, salt, and pepper in a bowl.

3.	Cut potato open and top with tuna salad and spinach.

4.	Enjoy!

Nutritional Information

- 350 calories

- 10g fat

- 40g carbs

- 25g protein

- 5g fiber

  - 300mg sodium

Serving Size: 1 baked potato

Prep Time: 10 minutes

8. Tuna Melt on Whole-Wheat English Muffin

Ingredients

- 2 slices whole-wheat English muffin
- 2 cans tuna in water, drained
- 1 tbsp low-fat mayonnaise
- 1 tsp Dijon mustard
- 1/4 cup chopped celery
- 1/4 cup shredded Swiss cheese

- Salt and pepper to taste

Preparation

1. Preheat broiler.

2. Combine tuna, mayonnaise, Dijon mustard, celery, salt, and pepper in a bowl.

3. Split and toast English muffins.

4. Top each muffin half with tuna salad and Swiss cheese.

5. Broil for 1-2 minutes, or until cheese is melted and golden brown.

6. Enjoy!

Nutritional Information

- 300 calories

- 10g fat

- 30g carbs

- 20g protein

- 2g fiber

- 350mg sodium

Serving Size: 1 open-faced sandwich

Prep Time: 10 minutes

9. Veggie Burger on a Whole-Wheat Bun

Ingredients

- 1 store-bought veggie burger patty
- Whole-wheat bun
- 1 lettuce leaf
- 1 tomato slice
- 1/4 cup sliced avocado
- 1 tbsp mustard
- 1 tsp ketchup

Preparation

1. Cook veggie burger patty according to package instructions.

2. Toast bun if desired.

3. Assemble burger with lettuce, tomato, avocado, mustard, and ketchup.

4. Enjoy!

Nutritional Information

- 350 calories

- 15g fat

- 30g carbs

- 20g protein

- 5g fiber

- 300mg sodium

Serving Size: 1 burger

Prep Time: 5 minutes

10. Chicken and Vegetable Soup with Brown Rice

Ingredients

- 4 cups chicken broth

- 1 Skinless chicken breast that is boneless , cooked and shredded

- 1 cup chopped carrots

- 1 cup chopped celery

- 1 cup chopped broccoli

- 1/2 cup chopped onion

- 1/2 cup cooked brown rice

- 1 tsp dried thyme

- Salt and pepper to taste

Preparation

1. Combine chicken broth, shredded chicken, carrots, celery, broccoli, onion, brown rice, and thyme in a pot.

2. Bring to a boil, then reduce heat and simmer for 15-20 minutes, or until vegetables are tender.

3. Add salt and pepper in order for it to taste

4. Enjoy!

Nutritional Information

- 300 calories

- 5g fat

- 40g carbs

- 25g protein

- 5g fiber

- 400mg sodium

Serving Size: 1 cup soup

Prep Time: 10 minutes

11. Turkey and Apple Salad with Walnuts

Ingredients

- 4 oz sliced turkey breast

- 1 apple, chopped

- 1/2 cup chopped celery

- 1/4 cup chopped walnuts

- 2 tbsp Greek yogurt

- 1 tsp lemon juice

- 1/2 tsp Dijon mustard

- Salt and pepper to taste

Preparation

1. Combine turkey, apple, celery, walnuts, Greek yogurt, lemon juice, Dijon mustard, salt, and pepper in a bowl.

2. Toss to combine and enjoy!

Nutritional Information

- 300 calories

- 10g fat

- 25g carbs

- 20g protein

- 5g fiber

- 250mg sodium

Serving Size: 1 salad

Prep Time: 10 minutes

12. Lentil and Vegetable Wraps with Hummus

Ingredients

- 1 cup cooked lentils
- 1/2 cup chopped carrots
- 1/2 cup chopped cucumber
- 1/4 cup chopped red onion
- 2 tbsp hummus
- 2 whole-wheat tortillas
- 1/4 cup chopped fresh parsley (optional)

Preparation

1. Combine cooked lentils, carrots, cucumber, red onion, hummus, and parsley (if using) in a bowl.

2. Spread hummus mixture onto whole-wheat tortillas.

3. Roll up tortillas and enjoy!

Nutritional Information

- 300 calories

- 5g fat

- 40g carbs

- 15g protein

- 5g fiber

- 250mg sodium

Serving Size: 1 wrap

Prep Time: 10 minutes

13. Salmon with Brown Rice and Roasted Vegetables

Ingredients

- 4 oz salmon fillet

- 1/2 cup cooked brown rice

- 1 cup chopped broccoli

- 1 cup chopped Brussels sprouts

- 1/2 cup chopped red onion

- 1 tbsp olive oil

- Salt and pepper to taste

Preparation

1. Preheat oven to 400°F (200°C).

2. Toss broccoli, Brussels sprouts, and red onion with olive oil, salt, and pepper.

3. Roast vegetables for 15-20 minutes, or until tender.

4. Season salmon with salt and pepper. Place on a separate baking sheet.

5. Bake salmon for 10-15 minutes, or until cooked through.

6. Serve salmon with brown rice and roasted vegetables.

Nutritional Information

- 350 calories

- 15g fat

- 30g carbs

- 30g protein

- 5g fiber

- 400mg sodium

Serving Size: 4 oz salmon fillet, 1/2 cup brown rice, and 1/2 cup roasted vegetables

Prep Time: 10 minutes

14. Tofu Scramble with Vegetables and Sprouts

Ingredients

- 1/2 block firm tofu, crumbled

- 1/2 cup chopped bell pepper (any color)

- 1/4 cup chopped onion

- 1/4 cup alfalfa sprouts

- 1/4 cup nutritional yeast

- 1 tbsp turmeric

- 1 tbsp paprika

- Salt and pepper to taste

- Olive oil spray

Preparation

1. Heat olive oil spray in a pan over medium heat.

2. Add onion and cook until softened.

3. Add bell pepper and cook for another 2-3 minutes.

4. Crumble tofu into the pan and cook until golden brown, stirring occasionally.

5. Stir in nutritional yeast, turmeric, paprika, salt, and pepper.

6. Cook for another minute or two, then stir in alfalfa sprouts.

7. Serve on whole-wheat toast or with a side of fruit.

Nutritional Information

- 250 calories

- 8g fat

- 20g carbs

- 20g protein

- 2g fiber

- 200mg sodium

Serving Size: 1/2 block tofu

Prep Time: 10 minutes

15. Black Bean and Mango Salad with Cilantro

Ingredients

- Black beans, drained and rinsed of 1 Can

- 1 mango, chopped

- 1/2 cup chopped red onion

- 1/4 cup chopped fresh cilantro

- 1 tbsp olive oil

- 1 tbsp lime juice

- Salt and pepper to taste

Preparation

1. Combine black beans, mango, red onion, cilantro, olive oil, lime juice, salt, and pepper in a bowl.

2. Toss to combine and enjoy!

Nutritional Information

- 250 calories

- 5g fat

- 35g carbs

- 10g protein

- 5g fiber

- 150mg sodium

Serving Size: 1 cup salad

Prep Time: 5 minutes

16. Quinoa Bowl with Roasted Vegetables and Tahini Dressing

Ingredients

- 1 cup cooked quinoa

- 1 cup chopped broccoli

- 1 cup chopped Brussels sprouts

- 1/2 cup chopped red onion

- 1 tbsp

- 1 tbsp olive oil

- Salt and pepper to taste

Tahini Dressing

- 2 tbsp tahini

- 1 tbsp lemon juice

- 1 tbsp water

- 1 clove garlic, minced

- Pinch of sea salt

Preparation

1. Preheat oven to 400°F (200°C).

2. Toss broccoli, Brussels sprouts, and red onion with olive oil, salt, and pepper.

3. Roast vegetables for 15-20 minutes, or until tender.

4. While vegetables roast, prepare tahini dressing by whisking together tahini, lemon juice, water, garlic, and salt until smooth.

5. Assemble quinoa bowls with cooked quinoa, roasted vegetables, and desired amount of tahini dressing.

6. Enjoy!

Nutritional Information

- 350 calories

- 10g fat

- 40g carbs

- 15g protein

- 5g fiber

- 300mg sodium

Serving Size: 1 bowl

Prep Time: 10 minutes

17. Chicken and Vegetable Power Bowl with Whole-Wheat Pita

Ingredients

- 4 oz grilled chicken breast, sliced

- 1 cup chopped romaine lettuce

- 1/2 cup chopped cucumbers

- 1/2 cup chopped tomatoes

- 1/4 cup chopped red onion

- 1/4 cup cooked brown rice

- 1/4 cup chickpeas, drained and rinsed

- 2 tbsp low-fat Greek yogurt

- 1 tbsp balsamic vinegar

- Salt and pepper to taste

- Whole-wheat pita bread

Preparation

1. Combine romaine lettuce, cucumbers, tomatoes, red onion, brown rice, chickpeas, and chicken in a bowl.

2. Whisk together Greek yogurt and balsamic vinegar to make a dressing.

3. The dressing should be poured over salad and tossed to combine.

4. Add salt and pepper for it to taste.

5. Serve with whole-wheat pita bread for scooping.

Nutritional Information

- 350 calories

- 5g fat

- 40g carbs

- 30g protein

- 5g fiber

- 300mg sodium

Serving Size: 1 bowl and 1/2 pita bread

Prep Time: 10 minutes

18. Turkey and Cranberry Salad with Spinach and Walnuts

Ingredients

- 4 oz sliced turkey breast

- 1 cup fresh spinach

- 1/2 cup chopped cranberries

- 1/4 cup chopped celery

- 1/4 cup chopped walnuts

- 2 tbsp light mayonnaise

- 1 tbsp lemon juice

- 1/2 tsp Dijon mustard

- Salt and pepper to taste

Preparation

1. Combine spinach, turkey, cranberries, celery, and walnuts in a bowl.

2. Whisk together mayonnaise, lemon juice, Dijon mustard, salt, and pepper in a small bowl.

3. The dressing should be poured over salad and toss to combine.

4. Enjoy!

Nutritional Information

- 300 calories
- 10g fat
- 25g carbs
- 20g protein
- 2g fiber
- 250mg sodium

Serving Size: 1 salad

Prep Time: 10 minutes

CHAPTER 3

Dinner Recipes

1. Baked Tilapia with Lemon and Herbs
Ingredients

- 4 tilapia fillets

- 1 tbsp olive oil

- 1/2 lemon, sliced

- 1 tsp dried thyme

- 1/2 tsp dried oregano

- Salt and pepper to taste

Preparation

1. Preheat oven to 400°F (200°C).

2. Place tilapia fillets on a baking sheet. Drizzle with olive oil and season with salt, pepper, thyme, and oregano.

3. Top each fillet with lemon slices.

4. Bake for 15-20 minutes, or until fish flakes easily with a fork.

Nutritional Information

- 250 calories

- 5g fat

- 35g protein

- 5g carbs

- 300mg sodium

Serving Size: 1 tilapia fillet

Prep Time: 5 minutes

2. Mediterranean Quinoa Bowl with Roasted Vegetables

Ingredients

- 1 cup quinoa, cooked

- 1 cup chopped broccoli

- 1 cup chopped Brussels sprouts

- 1/2 cup cherry tomatoes

- 1/4 cup chopped red onion

- 1 tbsp olive oil

- 1/2 lemon, juiced

- 1/4 cup crumbled feta cheese

- 1/4 cup chopped fresh parsley

- Salt and pepper to taste

Preparation

1.   Preheat oven to 400°F (200°C).

2.   Toss broccoli, Brussels sprouts, cherry tomatoes, and red onion with olive oil, salt, and pepper.

3.   Roast vegetables for 15-20 minutes, or until tender.

4.   Combine cooked quinoa, roasted vegetables, lemon juice, feta cheese, and parsley in a bowl.

5.   Add salt and pepper in order for it to taste

Nutritional Information

- 350 calories

- 10g fat

- 30g carbs

- 15g protein

- 5g fiber

- 300mg sodium

Serving Size: 1 bowl

Prep Time: 10 minutes

3. Salmon with Roasted Sweet Potato and Asparagus

Ingredients

- 4 salmon fillets

- 1 tbsp olive oil

- 1/2 teaspoon dried thyme

- Salt and pepper to taste

- 1 sweet potato, peeled and cubed

- 1 bunch asparagus, trimmed

Preparation

1. Preheat oven to 400°F (200°C).

2. Baking sheet should be lined with parchment paper.

3. On one half of the baking sheet, toss sweet potato cubes with olive oil, salt, and pepper. Spread into an even layer.

4. On the other half of the baking sheet, toss asparagus with olive oil, salt, and pepper. Spread into an even layer.

5. Place salmon fillets on top of the sweet potatoes. Season with olive oil, thyme, salt, and pepper.

6. Bake for 15-20 minutes, or until salmon is cooked through and vegetables are tender.

Nutritional Information

- 350 calories

- 15g fat

- 30g protein

- 20g carbs

- 5g fiber

- 350mg sodium

Serving Size: 1 salmon fillet with roasted vegetables

Prep Time: 10 minutes

4. Turkey Taco Lettuce Wraps

Ingredients

- 4 ground turkey patties, cooked and crumbled

- 4 large romaine lettuce leaves

- 1 cup chopped tomatoes

- 1/2 cup chopped cucumber

- 1/4 cup shredded red

- 1/4 cup black beans, drained and rinsed

- 1/4 cup salsa

- 1/4 cup chopped fresh cilantro

- 1 tbsp Greek yogurt

- 1 lime wedge

Preparation

1. Warm cooked ground turkey.

2. Assemble wraps by placing romaine lettuce leaves flat.

3. Spread each leaf with Greek yogurt.

4. Top with turkey, tomatoes, cucumber, red onion, black beans, and salsa.

5. It should be garnished with cilantro and a lime wedge.

Nutritional Information

- o 300 calories

- o 10g fat

- o 20g carbs

- o 25g protein

- o 5g fiber

- o 300mg sodium

Serving Size: 1 wrap

Prep Time: 10 minutes

5. Lentil and Vegetable Soup with Brown Rice

Ingredients

- 1 cup brown lentils, rinsed
- 4 cups vegetable broth
- 1 cup chopped carrots
- 1 cup chopped celery
- 1 cup chopped onion
- 1/2 cup chopped tomatoes
- 1 clove garlic, minced
- 1 tsp dried thyme
- 1/2 tsp dried oregano
- Salt and pepper to taste
- 1/2 cup cooked brown rice (optional)

Preparation

1. Combine lentils, broth, carrots, celery, onion, tomatoes, garlic, thyme, oregano, salt, and pepper in a pot.

2. Bring to a boil, then reduce heat and simmer for 30 minutes, or until lentils are tender.

3. Stir in cooked brown rice (if using).

4. Serve hot.

Nutritional Information

- 300 calories

- 5g fat

- 40g carbs

- 15g protein

- 5g fiber

- 400mg sodium

Serving Size: 1 cup soup

Prep Time: 10 minutes

6. Baked Chicken with Lemon and Herbs

Ingredients

- 4 bone-in, skinless chicken breasts

- 1 tbsp olive oil

- 1/2 lemon, juiced and zested

- 1 tsp dried thyme

- 1/2 tsp dried rosemary

- Salt and pepper to taste

Preparation

1. Preheat oven to 400°F (200°C).

2. Place chicken breasts in a baking dish.

3. It should be Drizzled with olive oil and season with salt, pepper, thyme, and rosemary.

4. Top with lemon juice and zest.

5. The chicken should be baked for 30-35 minutes, or until is cooked through.

Nutritional Information

- 300 calories

- 5g fat

- 40g protein

- 5g carbs

- 300mg sodium

Serving Size: 1 chicken breast

Prep Time: 10 minutes

7. Shrimp Scampi with Zucchini Noodles

Ingredients

- Raw shrimp, peeled and deveined of 1 pound
- 1 tbsp olive oil
- 2 cloves garlic, minced
- 1/2 cup dry white wine (optional)
- 1/4 cup chopped fresh parsley
- 1/4 cup lemon juice
- Salt and pepper to taste
- 2 zucchini, spiralized into noodles

Preparation

1. Olive oil should be heated in a large pan over medium heat.

2. Add garlic and cook until fragrant, about 30 seconds.

3. Add shrimp and cook until pink and cooked through, about 2-3 minutes per side.

4. If using, add white wine and simmer for 1 minute.

5. Stir in parsley, lemon juice, salt, and pepper.

6.	Add zucchini noodles and cook until heated through, about 1-2 minutes.

Nutritional Information

- 300 calories

- 5g fat

- 30g protein

- 5g carbs

- 2g fiber

- 400mg sodium

- **Serving Size:** 1 serving

- **Prep Time:** 10 minutes

8. Vegetarian Chili with Kidney Beans and Sweet Potato

Ingredients

- 1 tbsp olive oil
- 1 onion, chopped
- 2 cloves garlic, minced
- 1 bell pepper, chopped
- 1 (15 oz) can diced tomatoes
- 1 (15 oz) can kidney beans, drained and rinsed
- Black beans, drained and rinsed of 1 (15 oz)
- 1 sweet potato, peeled and diced
- 1 cup vegetable broth
- 1 tsp chili powder
- 1/2 tsp cumin
- 1/4 tsp smoked paprika
- Salt and pepper to taste

Preparation

1. Olive oil should be heated in a large pot over medium heat.

2.   Onions should be added and cooked until softened, about 5 minutes.

3.   Add garlic and bell pepper and cook for another 2-3 minutes.

4.   Add diced tomatoes, kidney beans, black beans, sweet potato, vegetable broth, chili powder, cumin, smoked paprika, salt, and pepper.

5.   Bring to a boil, then reduce heat and simmer for 30 minutes, or until sweet potato is tender.

Nutritional Information

- 350 calories

- 5g fat

- 45g carbs

- 15g protein

- 5g fiber

- 450mg sodium

Serving Size: 1 bowl

Prep Time: 15 minutes

9. Tuna Avocado Salad with Whole-Wheat Toast

Ingredients

- 2 cans tuna in water, drained

- 1 ripe avocado, mashed

- 1/2 lemon, juiced

- 1/4 cup chopped red onion

- 1/4 cup chopped celery

- 2 tbsp Greek yogurt

- 1 tsp Dijon mustard

- Salt and pepper to taste

- 2 slices whole-wheat toast

Preparation

1.   Combine tuna, avocado, lemon juice, red onion, celery, Greek yogurt, Dijon mustard, salt, and pepper in a bowl.

2.   Toast whole-wheat bread.

3.   Spread tuna avocado salad on toast and enjoy!

Nutritional Information

- 300 calories

- 15g fat

- 25g carbs

- 20g protein

- 5g fiber

- 300mg sodium

Serving Size: 2 open-faced sandwiches

Prep Time: 10 minutes

10. Chicken and Vegetable Stir-Fry with Brown Rice

Ingredients

- Boneless, skinless chicken breast of 1 pound, cut into strips

- 1 tbsp olive oil

- 1 onion, chopped

- 1 bell pepper, chopped

- 1 cup broccoli florets

- 1/2 cup chopped carrots

- 1/4 cup soy sauce

- 1 tbsp honey

- 1 tsp ginger paste

- 1/2 cup cooked brown rice

Preparation

1. Heat olive oil in a large pan or wok over medium-high heat.

2. Add chicken and cook until browned, about 5 minutes.

3. Add onion, bell pepper, broccoli, and carrots and cook for another 5-7 minutes, or until tender-crisp.

4. In a small bowl, whisk together soy sauce, honey, and ginger paste.

5. Pour sauce into the pan with the chicken and vegetables and cook for 1 minute, until heated through.

6. Serve over cooked brown rice.

Nutritional Information

- 350 calories
- 10g fat
- 30g carbs
- 30g protein
- 5g fiber
- 400mg sodium

Serving Size: 1 serving with brown rice

Prep Time: 10 minutes

11. Creamy Tomato Tortellini Soup with Spinach

Ingredients

- 1 tbsp olive oil

- 1 onion, chopped

- 2 cloves garlic, minced

- 1 (28 oz) can crushed tomatoes

- 4 cups vegetable broth

- 1 cup cooked cheese tortellini

- 1 cup baby spinach

- 1/2 cup low-fat milk or cream

- 1/4 cup grated Parmesan cheese

- Salt and pepper to taste

Preparation

1.   Olive oil should be heated in a large pot over medium heat.

2.   Onion should be added and cooked until softened, about 5 minutes.

3.   Garlic should be added and cooked for another minute.

4.   Add crushed tomatoes and vegetable broth.

5.   It should be brought to a boil, then reduce heat and simmer for 10 minutes.

6.   Add tortellini and spinach. Cook until tortellini is heated through and spinach is wilted, about 3-5 minutes.

7.   Stir in milk or cream and Parmesan cheese. Add salt and pepper in order for it to taste

8.   Serve hot.

Nutritional Information

- 300 calories

- 5g fat

- 40g carbs

- 15g protein

- 5g fiber

- 350mg sodium

Serving Size: 1 bowl

Prep Time: 10 minutes

12. One-Pan Lemon Garlic Chicken with Roasted Vegetables

Ingredients

- 4 boneless, skinless chicken breasts

- 1 tbsp olive oil

- 1/2 lemon, juiced and zested

- 1 tsp dried oregano

- 1/2 tsp salt

- 1/4 tsp black pepper

- 1 onion, chopped

- 1 bell pepper, chopped

- 1 cup broccoli florets

Preparation

1.   Preheat oven to 400°F (200°C).

2.   Toss chicken in olive oil, lemon juice and zest, oregano, salt, and pepper.

3.   Spread chicken in a single layer on a baking sheet.

4.   Surround chicken with chopped onion, bell pepper, and broccoli.

5.   Roast for 20-25 minutes, or until chicken is cooked through and vegetables are tender.

Nutritional Information

- 350 calories
- 10g fat
- 30g carbs
- 30g protein
- 5g fiber
- 400mg sodium

Serving Size: 1 chicken breast with roasted vegetables

Prep Time: 10 minutes

13. Grilled Salmon with Mango Salsa and Quinoa

Ingredients

- 4 salmon fillets

- 1 tbsp olive oil

- 1/2 lime, juiced

- 1/4 tsp salt

- 1/4 tsp black pepper

- 1 mango, chopped

- 1/4 cup red onion, chopped

- 1/4 cup chopped fresh cilantro

- 1 tbsp lime juice

- 1 cup cooked quinoa

Preparation

1.   Preheat grill to medium-high heat.

2.   In a bowl, toss salmon in olive oil, lime juice, salt, and pepper.

3.   In a separate bowl, combine mango, red onion, cilantro, and lime juice.

4.   Grill salmon for 4-5 minutes per side, or until cooked through.

5.   Serve salmon over cooked quinoa with mango salsa on top.

Nutritional Information

- 350 calories

- 15g fat

- 30g carbs

- 30g protein

- 5g fiber

- 350mg sodium

Serving Size: 1 salmon fillet with quinoa and mango salsa

Prep Time: 10 minutes

14. Curried Lentil and Sweet Potato Stew

Ingredients

- 1 tablespoon olive oil
- 1 onion, chopped
- 2 cloves garlic, minced
- 1 teaspoon ground ginger
- 1 teaspoon curry powder
- 1/2 teaspoon cumin
- 1/4 teaspoon turmeric
- 1 (14.5 oz) can diced tomatoes, undrained
- 4 cups vegetable broth
- 1 cup green lentils, rinsed
- Sweet potato, peeled and cubed
- 1 (15 oz) can chickpeas, drained and rinsed
- 1 cup chopped fresh spinach
- 1/2 cup chopped fresh cilantro
- Salt and pepper to taste
- Cooked brown rice or quinoa (optional)

Preparation

1. Olive oil should be heated in a large pot over medium heat.

2. Onions should be added and cooked until softened, for about 5 minutes.

3. Add garlic, ginger, curry powder, cumin, and turmeric. Cook for another minute, stirring constantly.

4. Add diced tomatoes and vegetable broth.

5. It should be brought to a boil after which you will reduce the heat and simmer for 10 minutes.

6. Stir in lentils, sweet potato, and chickpeas. The heat should be increased to medium-high and bring to a boil. Reduce heat, cover, and simmer for 20-25 minutes, or until lentils and sweet potato are tender.

7. Stir in spinach and cilantro. Cook for another minute, or until spinach is wilted.

8. Add salt and pepper in order for it to taste

9. Serve hot over cooked brown rice or quinoa, if desired.

Nutritional Information

- 350 calories

- 5g fat

- 50g carbs

- 15g protein

- 10g fiber

- 400mg sodium

Serving Size: 1 bowl

Prep Time: 10 minutes

CHAPTER 4

Snacks Recipes

1. Air-Popped Popcorn with Herbs and Spices

Ingredients

- 2 tbsp popcorn kernels

- 1 tsp olive oil

- 1/2 teaspoon dried thyme

- 1/4 teaspoon smoked paprika

- Salt and pepper to taste

Preparation

1. Combine olive oil, thyme, and paprika in a bowl.

2. Air-pop popcorn kernels.

3. Toss popcorn with the herb mixture. Season with salt and pepper.

Nutritional Information

- 150 calories

- 3g fat

- 25g carbs

- 3g protein

- 2g fiber

- 100mg sodium

Serving Size: 3 cups popcorn

Prep Time: 10 minutes (including popping time)

2. Edamame with Sea Salt and Lemon Zest

Ingredients

- o 1 cup frozen shelled edamame, thawed
- o 1/2 teaspoon sea salt
- o 1/4 teaspoon lemon zest

Preparation

- Steam or microwave edamame according to package instructions.
- Toss edamame with sea salt and lemon zest.

Nutritional Information

- 170 calories
- 8g fat
- 18g carbs
- 13g protein
- 3g fiber
- 300mg sodium

Serving Size: 1 cup

Prep Time: 5 minutes

3. Apple Slices with Almond Butter and Coconut

Ingredients

- o   1 apple, sliced

- o   2 tbsp almond butter

- o   1/4 cup unsweetened shredded coconut

Preparation

- Spread almond butter on apple slices. Sprinkle with coconut.

Nutritional Information

- 200 calories
- 8g fat
- 30g carbs
- 5g protein
- 5g fiber
- 100mg sodium

Serving Size: 1 apple with topping

Prep Time: 5 minutes

4. Roasted Chickpeas with Herbs and Spices

Ingredients

- 1 can chickpeas, drained and rinsed

- 1 tbsp olive oil

- 1/2 teaspoon dried rosemary

- 1/4 teaspoon cumin

- Salt and pepper to taste

Preparation

- Preheat oven to 400°F (200°C).
- Toss chickpeas with olive oil, rosemary, cumin, salt, and pepper.
- Spread chickpeas on a baking sheet and roast for 20-25 minutes, or until crispy.

Nutritional Information (per serving):

- 150 calories

- 3g fat

- 15g carbs

- 7g protein

- 5g fiber

- 150mg sodium

Serving Size: 1/2 cup chickpeas

Prep Time: 5 minutes

5. Yogurt Bark with Fruit and Nuts
Ingredients

- 1 cup plain Greek yogurt

- 1/4 cup mixed berries

- Chopped nuts (walnuts, almonds, etc.) of 1/4 cup

- 1 tbsp dark chocolate, chopped (optional)

Preparation

1. Baking sheet should be lined with parchment paper.

2. Yogurt should be spread evenly on the baking sheet.

3. Top with berries, nuts, and chocolate (if using).

4. Freeze for at least 2 hours, or until solid. Break into pieces and enjoy.

Nutritional Information

- 200 calories

- 5g fat

- 30g carbs

- 10g protein

- 2g fiber

- 200mg sodium

Serving Size: 4-6 pieces

Prep Time: 10 minutes

6. Roasted Sweet Potato Slices with Cinnamon and Sea Salt

Ingredients

- 1 medium sweet potato, thinly sliced

- 1 tbsp olive oil

- 1/2 teaspoon cinnamon

- Sea salt to taste

Preparation

1. Preheat oven to 400°F (200°C).

2. Toss sweet potato slices with olive oil and cinnamon.

3. Spread slices on a baking sheet and roast for 20-25 minutes, or until tender and crispy.

4. Sprinkle with sea salt before serving.

Nutritional Information

- 150 calories
- 3g fat
- 30g carbs
- 2g protein

- 3g fiber

- 100mg sodium

Serving Size: 1/2 sweet potato

Prep Time: 5 minutes

7. Carrot and Avocado Toast with Lemon Zest

Ingredients

- 1 slice whole-wheat bread

- 1/4 ripe avocado, mashed

- 1/4 cup grated carrot

- 1/4 teaspoon lemon zest

- Pinch of black pepper

Preparation

1. Toast whole-wheat bread.

2. Spread mashed avocado on toast.

3. Top with grated carrot and sprinkle with lemon zest and black pepper.

Nutritional Information

- 170 calories

- 6g fat

- 20g carbs

- 4g protein

- 3g fiber

- 100mg sodium

Serving Size: 1 slice toast

Prep Time: 5 minutes

8. Black Bean and Mango Salsa with Whole-Wheat Pita Chips
Ingredients

- Canned black beans of 1/2 cup, drained and rinsed

- 1/4 cup chopped mango

- 1/4 cup chopped red onion

- 1 tbsp chopped fresh cilantro

- 1 tbsp lime juice

- 1/4 teaspoon chili powder

- Pinch of salt and pepper

- Whole-wheat pita chips

Preparation

1. Combine black beans, mango, red onion, cilantro, lime juice, chili powder, salt, and pepper in a bowl.

2. Serve with whole-wheat pita chips.

Nutritional Information

- 150 calories

- 1g fat

- 30g carbs

- 5g protein

- 5g fiber

- 150mg sodium

Serving Size: 1/2 cup salsa with pita chips

Prep Time: 10 minutes

9. Greek Yogurt Smoothie with Banana and Spinach

Ingredients

- 1/2 cup plain Greek yogurt

- 1/2 banana

- 1/2 cup fresh spinach

- 1/4 cup unsweetened almond milk

- 1/4 teaspoon vanilla extract

- 1/2 cup ice (optional)

Preparation

1.   Blend all ingredients together until smooth. Add ice for a thicker consistency, if desired.

Nutritional Information

- 200 calories
- 5g fat
- 25g carbs
- 15g protein
- 3g fiber
- 150mg sodium

Serving Size: 1 smoothie

Prep Time: 5 minutes

10. Roasted Pumpkin Seeds with Herbs and Spices

Ingredients

- 1 cup pumpkin seeds
- 1 tbsp olive oil
- 1/2 teaspoon dried rosemary
- 1/4 teaspoon smoked paprika
- Salt and pepper to taste

Preparation

1.   Preheat oven to 400°F (200°C).

2.   Toss pumpkin seeds with olive oil, rosemary, paprika, salt, and pepper.

3.   Spread seeds on a baking sheet and roast for 10-15 minutes, or until golden brown and crispy.

Nutritional Information

- 150 calories

- 10g fat

- 5g carbs

- 5g protein

- 1g fiber

- 100mg sodium

Serving Size: 1/4 cup seeds

Prep Time: 5 minutes

CHAPTER 5

Desserts Recipes

1. Baked Cinnamon Apples with Berries

Ingredients

- 2 apples, cored
- 1/2 teaspoon cinnamon
- 1/4 cup mixed berries
- 1/4 cup chopped walnuts
- 1 tablespoon honey (optional)

Preparation

1. Preheat oven to 375°F (190°C).

2. Combine cinnamon and berries. Stuff apples with berry mixture.

3. Place apples in a baking dish and drizzle with honey (if using).

4. Bake for 25-30 minutes, or until apples are tender.

5. Top with chopped walnuts before serving.

Nutritional Information

- 150 calories

- 2g fat

- 35g carbs

- 2g protein

- 5g fiber

- 20mg sodium

Serving Size: 1 apple

Prep Time: 10 minutes

2. Dark Chocolate and Raspberry Mousse
Ingredients

- 1/2 cup plain Greek yogurt

- 3 tablespoons unsweetened cocoa powder

- 1/4 cup raspberries, mashed

- 1 tablespoon honey

- 1/4 cup chopped walnuts (optional)

Preparation

1.   In a bowl, whisk together yogurt, cocoa powder, mashed raspberries, and honey.

2.   Refrigerate for at least 2 hours, or until set.

3.   Top with chopped walnuts before serving (optional).

Nutritional Information

- 180 calories

- 5g fat

- 25g carbs

- 10g protein

- 2g fiber

- 60mg sodium

Serving Size: 1/2 cup

Prep Time: 10 minutes

3. Poached Pears with Honey and Yogurt

Ingredients

- 2 pears, peeled and cored

- 1 cup water

- 1/4 cup honey

- 1/4 cup plain Greek yogurt

- 1/4 teaspoon cinnamon

Preparation

1.   In a saucepan, combine water and honey. Bring to a simmer.

2.   Add pears and cook for 15-20 minutes, or until tender.

3.   Serve pears with yogurt and cinnamon.

Nutritional Information

- 170 calories

- 2g fat

- 40g carbs

- 5g protein

- 3g fiber

- 40mg sodium

Serving Size: 1 pear with yogurt topping

Prep Time: 5 minutes

4. Roasted Banana "Ice Cream" with Berries and Nuts

Ingredients

- 2 bananas, peeled and sliced
- 1/4 teaspoon cinnamon
- 1/4 cup mixed berries
- 1/4 cup chopped almonds

Preparation

1.   Preheat oven to 400°F (200°C).

2.   Toss banana slices with cinnamon and spread on a baking sheet.

3.   Roast for 15-20 minutes, or until softened and slightly browned.

4.   Top with berries and nuts.

Nutritional Information

- 180 calories

- 2g fat

- 40g carbs

- 2g protein

- 3g fiber

- 20mg sodium

Serving Size: 1 serving

Prep Time: 5 minutes

5. Watermelon and Mint Skewers with Honey Drizzle

Ingredients

- 1 cup cubed watermelon
- 10 mint leaves
- 1 tablespoon honey
- 1/4 teaspoon lime juice

Preparation

1. Thread watermelon cubes and mint leaves onto skewers.

2. Whisk together honey and lime juice. Drizzle over skewers.

Nutritional Information

- 50 calories
- 0g fat
- 12g carbs
- 0g protein
- 0g fiber
- 2mg sodium

- **Serving Size:** 4-5 skewers

- **Prep Time:** 5 minutes

6. Frozen Yogurt Bark with Berries and Nuts

Ingredients

- 1 cup plain Greek yogurt
- 1/4 cup mixed berries
- Chopped nuts (walnuts, almonds, etc.) of 1/4 cup
- 1 tablespoon dark chocolate, chopped (optional)

Preparation

1. Baking sheet should be lined with parchment paper.

2. Yogurt should be spread evenly on the baking sheet.

3. Top with berries, nuts, and chocolate (if using).

4. Freeze for at least 2 hours, or until solid. Break into pieces and enjoy.

Nutritional Information

- 200 calories
- 5g fat
- 30g carbs
- 10g protein
- 2g fiber
- 200mg sodium

Serving Size: 4-6 pieces

Prep Time: 10 minutes

7. Baked Apples with Oat Crumble

Ingredients

- 2 apples, cored

- 1/4 cup rolled oats

- 1/4 cup chopped walnuts

- 1/4 teaspoon cinnamon

- 1 tablespoon honey

Preparation

1. Preheat oven to 375°F (190°C).

2. Combine oats, walnuts, cinnamon, and honey.

3. Stuff apples with oat mixture.

4. Place apples in a baking dish and bake for 25-30 minutes, or until apples are tender and oat topping is golden brown.

Nutritional Information

- 200 calories

- 3g fat

- 40g carbs

- 5g protein

- 5g fiber

- 50mg sodium

Serving Size: 1 apple

Prep Time: 10 minutes

8. Chia Seed Pudding with Berries and Coconut

Ingredients

- 1/4 cup chia seeds

- 1 cup unsweetened almond milk

- 1/4 teaspoon vanilla extract

- 1/4 cup mixed berries

- 1/4 cup unsweetened shredded coconut

Preparation

1. Combine chia seeds, almond milk, and vanilla extract in a jar or bowl. Stir well and refrigerate overnight.

2. In the morning, top the pudding with berries and coconut.

Nutritional Information

- 250 calories

- 5g fat

- 35g carbs

- 8g protein

- 5g fiber

- 50mg sodium

Serving Size: 1 jar or bowl

Prep Time: 5 minutes (plus overnight refrigeration)

9. Greek Yogurt Parfait with Fruit and Granola

Ingredients

- o 1/2 cup plain Greek yogurt
- o 1/4 cup chopped fruit (mango, berries, etc.)
- o 1/4 cup granola

Preparation

1. Layer yogurt, fruit, and granola in a small bowl.

Nutritional Information

- 200 calories
- 5g fat
- 30g carbs
- 10g protein
- 2g fiber
- 200mg sodium

Serving Size: 1 small bowl

Prep Time: 5 minutes

10. Roasted Pears with Almond Butter and Pomegranate Seeds

Ingredients

- 2 pears, halved and cored
- 1 tablespoon almond butter
- 1/4 cup pomegranate seeds

Preparation

1. Preheat oven to 375°F (190°C).

2. Brush pears with almond butter.

3. Roast for 15-20 minutes, or until tender.

4. Top with pomegranate seeds before serving

Nutritional Information

- 180 calories
- 3g fat
- 35g carbs
- 4g protein
- 3g fiber
- 60mg sodium

- **Serving Size:** 1 pear half with topping

CHAPTER 6

7 DAYS MEAL PLAN

Day 1

Breakfast: Berry-licious Oatmeal with Chia Seeds & Nuts

Lunch: Mediterranean Tuna Salad Sandwich

Snack: Greek Yogurt Smoothie with Banana and Spinach

Dinner: Baked Tilapia with Lemon and Herbs

Day 2

Breakfast: Smoked Salmon & Avocado Whole-Wheat Toast

Lunch: Lentil Soup with Whole-Wheat Pita Bread

Snack: Air-Popped Popcorn with Herbs and Spices

Dinner: Mediterranean Quinoa Bowl with Roasted Vegetables

Day 3

Breakfast: Spinach & Egg Scramble with Tomatoes

Lunch: Salmon with Roasted Vegetables

Snack: Edamame with Sea Salt and Lemon Zest

Dinner: Salmon with Roasted Sweet Potato and Asparagus

Day 4

Breakfast: Overnight Oats with Berries and Nuts

Lunch: Chicken Caesar Salad with Whole-Wheat Croutons

Snack: Apple Slices with Almond Butter and Coconut

Dinner: Turkey Taco Lettuce Wraps

Day 5

Breakfast: Smoothie Bowl with Spinach, Banana & Peanut Butter

Lunch: Turkey and Avocado Wrap with Sprouts

Snack: Roasted Chickpeas with Herbs and Spices

Dinner: Lentil and Vegetable Soup with Brown Rice

Day 6

Breakfast: Cottage Cheese & Fruit Toast

Lunch: Black Bean and Corn Salad with Cilantro

Snack: Yogurt Bark with Fruit and Nuts

Dinner: Baked Chicken with Lemon and Herbs

Day 7

Breakfast: Scrambled Tofu with Bell Peppers and Onions

Lunch: Baked Potato with Tuna Salad and Spinach

Snack: Roasted Sweet Potato Slices with Cinnamon and Sea Salt

Dinner: Shrimp Scampi with Zucchini Noodles

CHAPTER 7

Conclusion

Congestive Heart Failure Cookbook for Seniors is an excellent resource for anyone dealing with the difficulties of maintaining their heart health. We have explored a variety of delicious and healthy dishes suited to address the special nutritional demands of seniors with congestive heart failure in this cookbook.

The emphasis on heart-healthy products, cautious portion control, and lower sodium intake is one recurring theme. These meals not only focus cardiovascular health, but they also highlight the gastronomic variety accessible in a heart-healthy diet. Seniors can actively maintain their heart health while still enjoying delectable meals by eating nutrient-rich foods such as lean meats, whole grains, and a range of fruits and vegetables.

Furthermore, the cookbook offers practical ideas and insights into choosing smart food choices, enabling elders to make long-term lifestyle improvements. The inclusion of nutritional information for each recipe allows users to make informed dietary choices and emphasizes the idea that tiny adjustments in eating habits can have a large influence on overall health.

As we come to the end of this culinary trip, keep in mind that living a heart-healthy lifestyle extends beyond the kitchen. A complete approach to heart health includes regular physical activity, proper hydration, and continuing communication with healthcare specialists. The Congestive Heart Failure Cookbook for Seniors is more than simply a cookbook; it's a guide to supporting long-term well-being.

Let these dishes serve as a starting point for a rich and satisfying journey in the spirit of greater heart health. Seniors can improve their quality of life and enjoy a heart-healthy culinary experience for years to come by embracing the principles stated in this cookbook.

THANKS FOR READING

www.ingramcontent.com/pod-product-compliance
Lightning Source LLC
Chambersburg PA
CBHW070950260726
48661CB00003B/1216